Crystal Wand Healing

ISBN 978-1-4710-6070-0

Hand of Light Publications

First Published in 2006

© Cover Design G-tigerclaw.com

email: healing@handoflight.org

website: www.handoflight.org

Dedicated to Fiona

...and everyone who helps to guide others towards their highest qualities of being

Richard was born in 1961 in Gloucestershire, England, UK. In 1966 his family moved to Leicestershire where Richard, together with his younger brother and sister, enjoyed a very creative childhood in countrified surroundings. It was here that he started building ride-in vehicles and inventing. He also became conscious of a spiritual side to his personality but was only able to identify it as such several years later.

In 1972 a move to Yorkshire continued the same environmental trend but a stressful secondary school existence caused emotional pain and stifled his enthusiasm. However, out of this experience he gained some significant spiritual awareness and in 1980, whilst away at college, began attending talks and workshops relating to spiritual development in order to discover and understand more.

In 1980, whilst living in Coventry, Richard took up the martial art of Kung-Fu and learnt about activating and using his 'Chi' energy. Applying what he learnt to his experiments in self-healing, and later combining this understanding with information from a library book on Crystal Power Tools, Richard discovered that healing both himself and various friends was actually very effective - speeding up the natural healing process several times over.

From 1985, Richard started to offer healing to close friends and noted their responses. In 1992 he moved to Bedfordshire and later ran evening classes in healing and weekend Crystal Wand-Making Workshops as part of an Adult Education programme. The Hand of Light website was established in 2003 and in its first 2 years attracted interest from 36 countries around the world.

Since 2005, Richard has given talks on healing and on using Crystal Wands. He is a firm believer in people taking responsibility for their own well-being and offers constructive support in personal empowerment to restore and maintain good health.

Contents

Section 2

A Hypothetical and Heuristic View of Healing

The importance of creating reality in relation to health

In the years ahead, people will have to learn to rely more on their own abilities to maintain good health - for themselves, their families, and their children. We all have to take personal responsibility for our own well-being and realise that we are the creative source of everything that happens to us in life.

Richard Gentle

Introduction

Illness and injury have become an accepted part of our lives. However, we can all do more to help ourselves and others gain an improvement in health or achieve complete recovery from illness.

I first came across the notion of healing people through non-medical means in the mid 1970's when reference was made to a family friend who 'did healing'.

Over the next several years, I read books, attended talks and workshops on spiritual development and generally started to 'have a go' myself. Among the things I became involved with along the way were: Kung-Fu; The Rosicrucians (AMORC); and a weekend workshop with an established healer, Matthew Manning. I later discovered a book on making Crystal Tools and began experimenting with a Crystal Wand.

By 2004 I had worked with people enduring every condition from minor injuries, aches and pains to more serious HIV, AIDS and Cancer. Some positive results exceeded expectation while others left me wondering what was going on! However, I can now offer an explanation, albeit in part a somewhat controversial one.

This book is divided into two sections. Section one keeps things simple and tells you how to make, cleanse, and use a Crystal Wand. Section two is more advanced and looks at the whole process of healing in more detail. This includes exploring some aspects of the universe that are still to be fully understood.

We will look at some of the reasons why injury and illness serves us and show that, through a change in mental approach to our circumstances and developing an understanding of using the Crystal Wand in combination with Personal Action Intervention, we can learn to take more responsibility for our own health and well-being.

SECTION ONE

Common Health Cycles

Let's begin by looking at some of the health cycles most familiar to us.

Physical Injury
- A physical injury occurs
- All mental attention is focused on the area of pain
- Breathing rate increases
- Our pain is expressed verbally by cursing or crying
- We rub or grip the injured area with a hand

General Illness
- We hear that an ailment is 'going around'
- We catch a cold
- We feel debilitated for days or weeks

Serious Disease
- We feel under stress - worries about life or relationships, a traumatic experience, or guilt from reckless behaviour
- Emotional transference - upset leading to physical illness
- We may or may not recover

Why?
There are many reasons why people suffer injury or illness. There are also many symptoms whose causes may not at first seem clear. I was once told that our natural state is one of health, but no one really explained what that meant and why so many of us become afflicted with such a variety of ailments. Over time, I have realised the truth of this statement and come to understand its amazing message: You can choose to be well.

If you read the whole of this book, you will find more in-depth information on how constant good health can be maintained.

Crystal Wands

There are several different types of wand and wand design but I am only going to focus on one. The crystal wand I am going to discuss is not a single shard of crystal (often referred to as a wand) and it is not a solid stick of wood with a crystal at the end. It is also not a crystal at the end of a tube filled with other material. The crystal wand I am going to be using is not overly embellished and it is not derived from Shamanic origins or Earth Magic.

The basic wand consists of a copper tube with a clear quartz crystal in one end and a solid blank end-cap at the opposite end. The wand is bound with leather (a non-conductive fabric can be used for those who prefer not to use animal skins). Some believe that this type of wand has its origin in the ancient lost city of Atlantis, but I cannot comment on the truth of this.

Once the assembly of the wand is completed, it has to be cleansed and programmed before first use. You will then have a very powerful and effective light/energy tool to help with healing.

Amazing Properties and Qualities of Crystal Wands
During the time I have used wands, I have noticed the following:

- The crystal wand is self-cleansing in sunlight
- The crystal wand has antiseptic actions on infected wounds
- The crystal wand is exceptionally effective on aches, sprains, bone aches, and rheumatism
- The crystal wand speeds up the normal healing process
- Use of the crystal wand is 'non-invasive'
- Energy from the crystal wand automatically goes to where it is needed within the area of focus
- The healing effects from the crystal wand can continue for some days after treatment

Misunderstandings
Used correctly, the wand will not absorb and harbour energy from a client, thus it is safe to use between clients. The nature of use is one of projecting energy out rather than 'drawing it in'.

Because leather is from an animal, some believe that its 'lower vibrational energy' affects the purity of the wand and its ability to be used in healing. Whilst this view may prevail in some applications employing animal-derived products, it does not apply in the case of the wand. The wrapping of the wand in non-conductive material has a very specific purpose of insulating physical contact from the copper shaft. (Leather does not have to be used - it simply has a nice feel to many, is a traditional material, and offers good durability). I will only add that it is important that you feel comfortable with your wand and you should therefore select materials that you feel comfortable using.

Selecting a Crystal
For this type of healing wand you need to use a clear quartz crystal. These are readily available although they will vary in price. The cost of the crystal is not important but ideally you should select something with good undamaged face edges. Also, the crystal should be reasonably clear and possibly contain rainbows or interesting reflections and patterns. Hold the crystal in your hand and notice any feeling or impressions you receive from it. For example:

- Does the crystal make you feel good?
- Does the crystal sparkle with vitality and life?
- Does the crystal seem to contain and reflect a vibrant light as you move it around?

Making a Crystal Wand
You will need to obtain the following materials and tools:

Materials
- 12 inch length of copper tubing 22 millimetres diameter
- One copper end-cap to fit 22mm tube
- One Quartz Crystal approximately 1½ to 2 inches long with a diameter slightly larger than the diameter of the tube
- A length of leather (or non-conductive material of your choice) approximately 1 inch wide and 4 feet long (or enough to wrap the length of the wand shaft)
- Solder
- Double-sided sticky tape
- Hot-weld glue or epoxy resin glue

Tools
- Pen, pencil, scissors
- Hacksaw with metal-cutting blade
- Small metal files
- Fine abrasive paper
- Hot-weld Glue-Gun (unless using resin-based epoxy glue)
- Small bench vice
- Gas Blow-torch
- Pliers

Construction
Refer to the diagrams and instructions over the next few pages. When clamping the wand in the bench vice it is sensible to place some material between the wand and the jaws of the vice to avoid damaging the wand.

- Cut the copper tube to exactly 12 inches in length (use a pipe cutter for best results or file edges after sawing)
- Clean one end with abrasive paper around the area that the end cap will cover

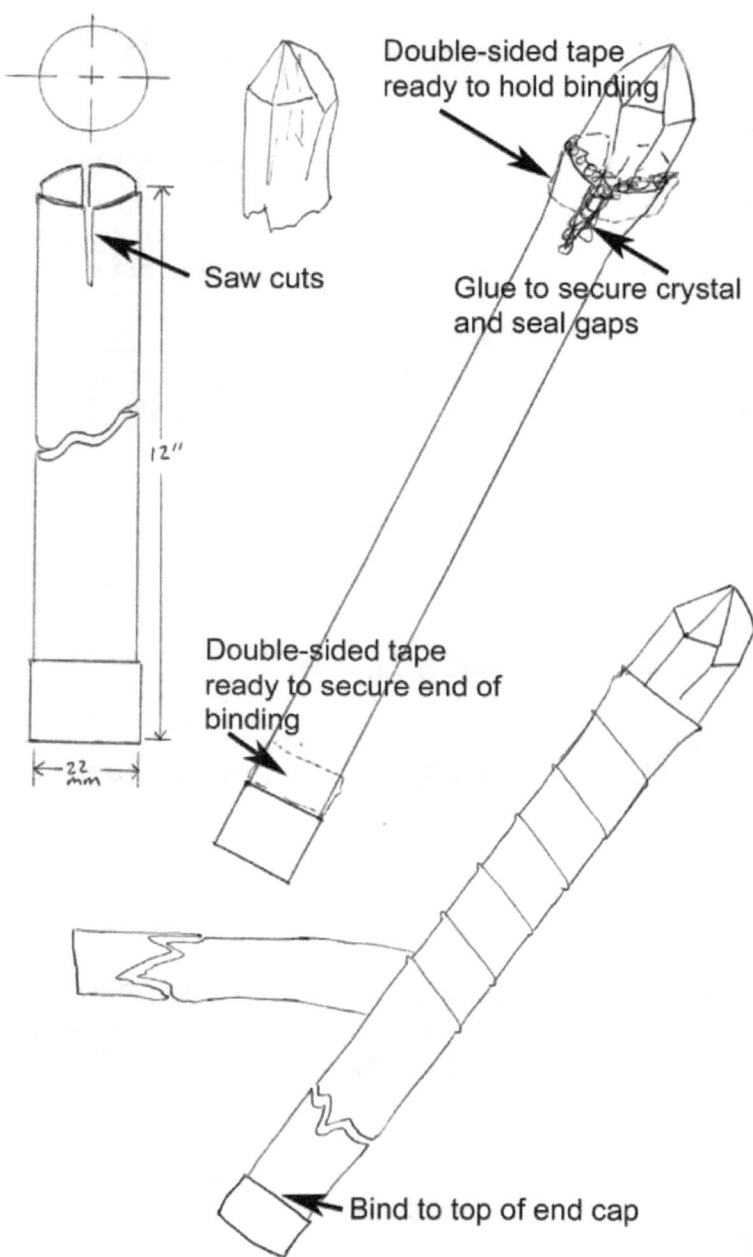

Saw cuts

Double-sided tape ready to hold binding

Glue to secure crystal and seal gaps

12"

22 mm

Double-sided tape ready to secure end of binding

Bind to top of end cap

- Clamp the tube horizontally in the bench vice. Push the end cap onto the tube and heat the area with the blow-torch. When hot, run some solder around the joint
- Carefully remove the tube (it will be red hot) and quench it in a sink of cold water (or run tap water over it). Do not let water get into the tube.
- File or smooth off any excess lumps of solder
- Place the tube in the vice and using a hack saw, cut a cross about ¾ of an inch deep at the open end of the tube. File any rough edges and tip the filings out of the wand
- Use the pliers to bend the open end of the tube to form a clasp for the crystal. The crystal should be held loosely. Try to get the crystal to rest as centrally and as vertically as possible. Keep removing the crystal, modifying the clasp and replacing the crystal - until you get a good fit.
- Check the clasp for any new rough edges and file as necessary. Remember to empty the filings from the tube
- Run some glue around the inside top edges of the clasp and quickly place the crystal - try to maintain alignment
- Once the first glue has set and the crystal is held, continue to put glue around the areas where the crystal meets the clasp. Seal any gaps with glue to make sure water cannot enter the tube later (in the cleansing process)
- Wrap some double-sided tape around both ends of the tube (see diagram) but leave the top protective cover in place
- Cut a length of leather or chosen material (see previous description in 'materials'). Practise getting the wrap angle correct before exposing the double-sided tape. You will also need to trim the end of the leather before starting the wrap. (Where to trim will become obvious during your initial practise).
- Uncover the double-sided tape (at the crystal end) and wrap the leather from the crystal end down to the bottom of the wand shaft - finishing level with the start of the end-cap. You need to wrap the leather at an angle down the wand so that it overlaps slightly as you move along.

Pull the leather very tightly, wrap around, pull tightly, wrap around, etc. As you get to the last wrap before securing the end of the leather, relax the tightness so that the leather isn't going to pull off the double-sided tape. Trim the leather so that the last wrap follows the correct line and then remove the cover from the tape and secure the leather in place. (You may have to add a little more tape, or use some suitable glue to fully fix the end of the wrap).

Cleansing and Programming
Before a wand is used for the first time, it has to be cleansed, programmed, and activated.

Cleansing
It is important to cleanse the quartz crystal wand of any negative energy vibrations that it may have picked up or accumulated before first use. After the first cleansing and programming, the wand will be self-cleansing when left in sunlight.

There are a few ways to cleanse wands. My recommendation for cleansing healing wands is to use fresh flowing water. A location such as a river, waterfall, or a reservoir with some wave motion is ideal. Wherever you decide to go, try to make it a place which is either special to you personally, or where you feel there is a natural and powerful Earth energy centre. Ideally, wait until you have a sunny day and preferably go out in the morning while the sun is still rising.

Programming
It is important to program your wand with the intention you have for its use. This will ensure that directed energy is specific and not confused.

Dip the end of the wand into the water so that only the crystal is fully submerged. As you hold the wand there, say the following words aloud (or inside your head):

'I cleanse this crystal wand of all impurity and program it for the use of healing and amplification of positive intention.'

(You may use your own wording if you prefer, so long as the essence of what you say is positive and of similar intention to the above).

Remove the wand from the water and allow it to dry naturally in the air - do not dry it with a cloth etc.

If the sun is shining, you can also hold the wand to the sky, and towards the sun, and repeat the words you used whilst the wand was in the water. All of this reinforces your intention for the way the wand will be used.

Storage
The best place to keep your wand when not in use is on a windowsill facing east. (Face north if East is not possible). The reason for facing east is because this is where the sun rises and the day is renewed. Wands like to be in the sunlight but any natural daylight is okay.

Transportation
Wrap the wand in a soft cloth (velvet or similar material is ideal) so that when it is being transported, the faces of the crystal are not damaged.

Using your wand
Before using your wand for the first time, it is useful to perform the following exercises. If you are already familiar with what follows, you will already know why these exercises are helpful.

As you get used to using the wand, you will not need to go through these exercises. You will simply point the wand towards the target area for healing and see the light and healing energy emanating from the wand and out towards the area to be healed.

Using the wand is straightforward, but to be an effective practitioner, you really need to know about some of the background details and techniques.

Exercises

Exercise 1 - Thumb Squeeze
- Squeeze one of your thumbs with your other hand
- Hold the squeeze for 20 seconds
- Let go and try to continue feeling the thumb that was squeezed without actually touching it

Exercise 2 - Breathing
- Breathe in through the nose and out through the mouth. (If you find it difficult to breathe through your nose, your mouth will be okay)
- Breathe deeply from the diaphragm
- Imagine breathing in at the bottom, the top, and in the middle. (Don't worry about the reality of this, it's just a way to ensure you think about filling your lung capacity)

If you start to feel a little light-headed, stop for a while and allow normal stability to return before having another go.

What does breathing do?
In addition to oxygenating the blood supply, it focuses the attention. Add a word or two in your mind on the out breath (exercise 5) and your concentration becomes incredibly focused.

Exercise 3 - Combination
- Repeat exercise 1
- As soon as you let go of the thumb, do the breathing exercise 2 (above)
- As you breathe out, focus your attention on the thumb that was squeezed (without physically touching it)

You should notice that the length of time you can feel the squeezed thumb has become extended.

Exercise 4 - Sending Energy
Using the same techniques as previously described, have a go at sending energy to other areas of your body. As you breathe out, focus your attention and see if you can feel a sensation in any area you focus on.

Exercise 5 - Adding Words
Repeat the last exercise but this time as you breathe out, say [inside your mind] the words 'cleanse and heal'.

Exercise 6 - Seeing Light (Fingers Exercise)
Touch the fingertips of both hands together and slowly pull them apart. See if you can notice lines of light still joining the fingertips together between the two hands. This exercise probably works best against a dark background - you may see silvery threads.

Exercise 7 - Simple Sunlight Technique
Usually, while I am physically present and healing someone, I often give him/her a little exercise to do. However, this exercise can be used by anyone at any time, day or night:

Imagine bright morning sunlight shining down on you. Imagine the sunlight shining on your head. Feel the sunlight and its warmth. As you breathe in, take the sunlight down through the top of your head. As you breathe out, imagine the light going to any area of your body where you want healing to take place.

Exercise 8 - Playing with Finger Light
Perform exercise 7 but this time as you breathe out imagine sending the sunlight that is now inside you, around your body, down one of your arms, and into your hand. Imagine that the light keeps going until it starts to come out of your fingers. Pretend that you can see light flowing out of you. (With a little practice and patience, you may find you can actually see something).

Healing with your Hands

Using the techniques described in the exercises, start to practise your healing. The easiest way to begin is by having a go on yourself or a friend - perhaps the next time you or they have a minor cut, an ailment, or an injury.

Point your index finger at the injured area and send healing energy down your arm and out of your finger towards the injured area. Imagine healing energy and light leaving your finger and surrounding the injured area. You can try the same technique using your whole hand - imagining healing energy and light leaving your palm and massaging the injured area.

Using the Wand

Now that you are familiar with the basic exercises and the projection of energy to areas of your body through mental focus and breath control, it is simply a matter of introducing the crystal wand into the equation.

Exercise 9 - Activating the Wand

Hold the wand in your hand (left or right) and when you breathe out, send energy down your arm, into your hand and then from your hand into the Wand. Imagine the energy activating the Wand like a flash tube around a ruby laser.[1] As you breathe in, charge yourself up. As you breathe out, send energy into the Wand.

Exercise 10 - Wand Light

Pick up your wand and hold it in a relaxed grip with your hand - approximately in the middle of its length. Now repeat exercise 9 but this time, when you send the light to your hand, project it into the wand and out through the crystal.

---

[1] See description of Ruby Laser in Section 2

Removing Yourself

Exercise 11 - Energy from the Universal Energy Field
This exercise focuses healing energy directly from the sentient field, through the wand, to the client. It's a good way to ensure that you do not cause interference by channelling through your own body and also prevents you from becoming tired or affected by changes in your own energy.

Hold the wand as described above (exercise 10) and this time try visualising vibrant energy from all around you entering the blanked end of the Wand. The electrons[2] are excited by your grip around the Wand and photons[3] begin to be produced, exiting the Wand through the crystal in a stream of light.

Focus your attention on the crystal and as you breathe out, see light and healing energy coming out of the wand. With practice you will be able to see the energy.

Mastery of the Wand
You hold the wand a few inches from the client and move from head to toes through the etheric field - first down one side and then repeating the process again down the other side.

You aim the wand an inch or two from the client in the area being healed and focus your attention and breathing. You see light energy streaming from the wand and into the client. You no longer have to think about the process. You simply know that the healing is working and you expect to gain an improvement in health for the person receiving the healing.

---

[2] Electron - Elementary particle with negative charge
[3] Photon or light particle - A quantum of electromagnetic radiation

The Crystal Wand Healing Experience

"Over the past three years, I have received repeated abnormal smear results of type CN3 - severe abnormal cell changes - treated by various means of surgery.

In August last year, I returned from a holiday to France with acute stomach pains. My GP suspected gallstones and prescribed medication and antacids. Some ten days later, barely able to eat or sleep, I received Crystal Wand healing for the first time. The result was both remarkable and completely unexpected. Instantly, the pain abated and to this day has never recurred. I subsequently received healing on other occasions to successfully alleviate migraine headaches.

By now, having experienced the healing potential of the wand, I was curious as to the effect this may have on the abnormal cell changes that kept recurring. A couple of months prior to my next smear I received a course of healing focussing on this area. I was staggered and overjoyed when the result came back negative - my first all clear result in over 3 years. As no other variable had changed during this period, such as diet and lifestyle, I am firmly convinced that the healing was wholly responsible. I have since had my own wand made and wand myself regularly as a means of maintaining good health."

Amelia, West Yorkshire

"I was suffering from a bout of bursitis in my shoulder [bursitis causes inflammation and pain around joints, tendons, and ligaments]. Pain killers were of little help. However, after only two Crystal Wand healing sessions the acute pain dissipated.

On another occasion, I had a severe toothache and after one session, the pain had gone in a matter of hours.

At first I was sceptical, but do believe that the Crystal Wand healing definitely helped. I could feel the energy emitted from the wand. It was like cool air brushing up against my skin or like placing your hand in proximity of a negative ionising device."

George, South Yorkshire

"I've always seen myself as rational, not influenced by things mystical. Working with students in the late sixties, surrounded by dope, LSD and the I-Ching - I remained unscathed. When Richard first talked about crystal healing, I was interested, but sceptical. Our German shepherd dog suffered from arthritis in her back legs, and it seemed a good test, because I couldn't see any way a placebo effect could work on a dog. Although Richard's wand didn't cure her, it did seem to give her some relief during her remaining years.

Then my partner who is a professional musician, playing keyboards, developed an arthritic thumb, which worried him. Richard did some healing with him and he felt immediately better. I decided to explore this and asked Richard to make me a wand. He gave me instructions for preparing the crystal. I was happy with the cleansing aspect in a mountain stream, but less convinced by the words I was supposed to use. But I did it. When I came to use the wand, I had no idea of any special things to do or think, so I just held it and moved it slightly around my partner's thumb in ways I'd seen Richard do it. To our complete surprise it worked. I should explain that my partner is of a scientific bent and pre-disposed to scoff. He says it shouldn't work, but it does.

Last summer, a friend cut his finger badly on a very sharp knife. We tried the wand and he reported that it felt as if his finger was being healed from the inside. In a very few days it was completely healed. Normally I'd expect a cut this deep to leave a scar, but there was none.

A few weeks ago, my doc told me I had what he called a "small hernia". I've been using my own wand, supplemented by a few sessions from Richard. I can't claim that the hernia has been cured yet, but the doc said it would get worse, which it hasn't done. It certainly feels less uncomfortable than it did.

I think the crystal works better on some problems than on others, and you discover what works well by experiment. The issue of the placebo effect is always raised as a possibility, but I don't think that matters if you get better. Maybe what's happening is that the wand helps you to feel you are taking charge for your own healing? I don't think it matters how it works, what's important is that it works for you."

Dave, West Yorkshire

SECTION TWO

A Hypothetical and Heuristic View of Healing

This section of the book briefly touches on and explores a number of other areas connected with healing.

Different Illness
It's perhaps tempting to divide illness into categories such as physical and mental, etc., but in universal actuality there is no absolute differentiation here. Later, I will focus on some of the origins of illness and some of its manifestations in physical form. For now, I will focus only on physical injury and illness. This approach demonstrates best, the approach you need to adopt in maintaining good health.

Physical Injury
Let's begin by looking at the process that occurs when we receive a physical injury. Let's take an example of accidentally stubbing your toe on something hard.

1. You feel the onset of pain where you have been injured.
2. You might shout out or cry
3. You grab your foot with your hand in an attempt to stem the pain
4. Your breathing and heart rate increases
5. All your attention becomes focused on your injury
6. After a while the toe begins to throb and you may feel heat around the injured area
7. Gradually the pain diminishes
8. Over time, the toe returns to its former healthy state

So, now that we have dissected the event, let's deliberately go through the actions as if we have all hurt ourselves in the way mentioned above, only this time we manage our response differently:

1. The pain tells you something has happened and in this example, where it is
2. As you hold the injured area, you control your breathing and slow it down. As you breathe out, you control the speed of your exhalation and blow slowly with some pressure [through pursed lips].
3. You imagine healing energy travelling to the injured area
4. You release your grip on the foot and point a finger at your toe - about an inch away
5. You repeat your breathing exercise and project healing energy from your finger into the toe
6. Although you can feel the toe throbbing, you accept this as feedback that the healing process has begun
7. The pain gradually subsides
8. The toe recovers rapidly over a very short time

Physical Illness

The way in which a body becomes weakened or damaged, due to any number of ailments or diseases, is very interesting. Illness can begin from a simple suggestion, right through to very complex experiences and circumstances. Unlike physical injury, physical illness and disease (with little damage showing on the surface) is sometimes more difficult to come to terms with. When you scratch the skin or break a bone, somehow everything is more tangible. When you have something like a cold or a cancer, it's often more difficult to see, know, or understand what is going on. It is somehow in our comprehension to watch a visible wound heal and form a scar, but beyond our understanding when something hidden from our physical vision seems to march on relentlessly - ravaging us and eroding our very existence and quality of life from within.

Getting Started

To get started with healing, you need to understand something of the nature of your own being and the creative energy within you.

Illness is often perceived as a serious issue for those suffering - whether it be the individual with the illness, or a partner, parents, children, relatives, friends, or associates. However, if you want to see improvements in health, it is important to have a broader understanding of why illness may have arisen and to then see how it may be reversed - or ideally, prevented from occurring in the first place. Many of us now appreciate that treating symptoms does not always heal causes. Treat the causes and you alleviate or reverse the symptoms. And when I say 'treat the causes', I am not referring here only to perceived physical causes.

The Conventional Spiritual View

Some people attribute their well-being - or lack of it - to certain beliefs they have developed. Sometimes, if we suffer persistent illness, we might have cause to wonder if we have done something wrong in our life... but not just our current life - our past lives! The concept of reincarnation has been around for a long time. Although traditionally more accepted in eastern religions and cultures, it nevertheless has caused some people to think more broadly about their existence and wonder whether there is a balance of deeds done that exists throughout time. Unfortunately, holding rigidly to this view may prevent a person from moving forward and realising his/her full potential in the life that he/she is now experiencing.

Karma

Karma is an essentially eastern construct about cause and effect. Some people believe that for every action committed in life, particularly against another sentient being, there is an action of retribution similar to the act committed. By behaving in a considerate manner towards all things, a person can keep his/her Karma in balance and even improve his/her future life or lives. Even in science there is a belief that 'for every action, there is an equal and opposite reaction'. Commonly, other expressions such as: 'What goes around comes around', is a view many cultures comfortably embrace.

However, there is a tendency to use the expression as a qualifier to a deed you have done which you consider 'good' and deserving of reward or conversely, 'bad' and deserving of some punishment. Furthermore, the concept of Karma is used by some people to make them feel better when they judge that someone has done a 'bad' deed against them. When someone else deserves a punishment that you are unable to bestow, at least you can comfort yourself by believing it will surely come to them by 'other means'. In all cases people actively seek retribution on their terms of judgement.

There are many stories in life where people have participated in an activity or event and moments or years later, have been on the receiving end of an apparently parallel experience. Some people believe that such experiences can spread across several reincarnate lifetimes until a point of resolution is reached for all concerned.

In the Jane Roberts[4] books, Seth[5] tells us that reincarnate lives exist simultaneously so there is constant give-and-take between them. A future life can affect a past one as much as a past one can affect a present one, so karma as it is usually considered does not apply. Seth also says that karma does not involve punishment. "Karma presents the opportunity for development. It enables the individual to enlarge understanding through experience, to fill gaps of ignorance, to do what should be done. Free will is always involved".[6] Seth later continues [in the same book]: "A problem is a challenge set up by the entity for one of its own personalities, but the outcome is up to the personality involved".

One reason for our expectation of retribution is connected to our feelings of compassion and ideas about guilt. We create the circumstances for our own resolutions.

---

[4] Jane Roberts - Channel and author of the Seth books
[5] The Nature of Personal Reality
[6] The Seth Material

The Etheric Body and Aura

From a conventional spiritual viewpoint, the human body is broadly composed of two parts. The physical body - which is sometimes called the dense or corporeal body, and the etheric body - which is called various things - the etheric double, the vital-body, the energy body, the bioplasmic body, or the aura. (The term 'aura', is generally used to describe a visual aspect of the etheric body - usually visible to those sensitive enough to see it (a skill that can be developed in varying degrees by most people), or by those using equipment that can detect it).

The etheric body permeates the physical body and is essentially the real energy of what you are. Some believe that the etheric body stores information on such things as, the root causes and state of physical, emotional and mental imbalances. Within the etheric body are energy centres called chakras. These control many of our physical, mental, psycho-emotional and spiritual states. The chakras often go 'out of balance' due to our often unbalanced lifestyles, but they are also usefully activated in various ways when practising healing. (Chakras are of course activated at other times - not necessarily only when healing). Chakras are sometimes described as spinning wheels of energy.

That Sudden Jolt

Sometimes, the etheric body moves slightly out of alignment with the physical body. Most people have a direct experience of this happening when becoming drowsy - a sudden noise or stray thought that brings you back to full consciousness with a jolt. This is the etheric body snapping back into alignment again with the physical body.

A further extension of this effect can be developed into a technique called astral projection, but this is not an area I am going to look at here. In its most common form, this slight misalignment allows us to recharge the body's vitality - in layman's terms, a good rest or good night's sleep.

It is not my intention to go into exhaustive detail here (there are many books and web sites that can give more information for those who wish to gain a deeper understanding), suffice to say it is useful to have awareness of the etheric body when practising healing. Most often, it is 'damage' to the etheric body that then manifests as illness or disease in the physical body. To heal the physical effectively, you must first heal the etheric. Be aware too, that the way we think affects the health of our etheric body.

Colour

Colour is a very useful aspect of healing to know about. For the purposes of this book, I am only going to mention two colours: blue and red. The blue is good for healing and the red is good for boosting energy levels. The blue should be a vibrant mid-blue and the red should also be vibrant - like the colour of a traditional British mail box.

Music

Sometimes, it is more relaxing for the client if some gentle music is playing in the background whilst healing is taking place. Music should be fairly innocuous and consistent in overall volume level with no sudden changes. Sounds from nature or a composition of calmness are ideal.

Visualisation

Many people are familiar with the concept of visualisation. Imagination - pictures and sensations in the mind, affecting your mood and your body - can also be projected from you to others - can be released into the universe. What you may not realise is that we visualise all of the time - not just when we consciously choose to visualise (perhaps through meditation or daydreaming). And very often, what we visualise most is what 'plays' on our mind - such as when we worry about something.

Some research mentioned in the book and film, 'What the "Beep" do we know?' points to evidence that brain function of an actual experience is identical to when we recall that experience just by thinking about it again. This prompts the question: 'How do we know what is real?'

Healing Squared
There is a widely held view among people involved with spiritual healing that the more people you can get involved, the better. When one person sends healing, that is one person. When two people send healing, the ratio is squared, thus four people effectively send healing. Ten people sending healing would be like one hundred people sending healing.

The Progressive View

Unaware Visualisations
Unaware visualisations can include 'self-talk'. Okay, we know what we are saying, but perhaps we don't consciously hear what we are saying. Consider the following:

- How we talk to ourselves (self-talk) affects our reality - we affirm our condition and our physical mood reflects this
- What we think about affects our reality - focus instigating probable events[7]
- What we say out loud also affects our reality - regardless of being alone or with others
- What other people say to us can affect our reality - if we decide to let it influence our thinking

What we think and say is what we end up believing. What we believe becomes manifest in our experience of physical reality. When we focus on a thought we begin to feel the reality of what we are creating. This feeds back into our creative visualisation and intensifies the resultant feeling. As we progress in this fashion we start to manifest a physical experience of our belief. Once we have a physical result this becomes solid proof of our

---

[7] Every thought produces or modifies a possible outcome or 'probable event'.

situation. And when this happens it can be difficult to reverse the process in the face of the 'hard physical evidence'.

Media Bombardment
A constant flow of negative news reports and images feeds our conscious minds and colours our view of the world. Sometimes we resonate with elements transmitted to us because they fit our existing beliefs about the world. These elements go into our unconscious thoughts and feelings. Most of us are influenced by something and like a superstition we hold onto some notions more than others. These embed themselves in our unconscious imagination and we behave as though they exist in our sense of reality.

Some examples of this include:
- Anti-smoking campaigns with cigarette packets showing such labels as, 'Smoking Kills' rather than something like, 'Stop Smoking'
- News items warning of illness epidemics, problems with some foods, and increases in violence, etc. rather than focusing on noticeable improvements in well-being

In each case, these messages enter our unconscious processes via our conscious mind. It is often difficult to ignore these messages, portrayed as they are, with dramatic emphasis and visually stimulating imagery. Our minds feed on things that impress us, stand out from the crowd, or indulge our fixation for worrying.

Another example of how we are affected by this sort of media bombardment is fuel shortages. The message, 'Don't panic-buy' is a sure way to get people to do just that! Without the message, people carry on as normal and any fuel shortage is hardly noticed and soon rectified. Likewise, the message that, 'many people are likely to die from a new disease', affects a population who then keeps looking to see if they are developing symptoms. People 'expect' to be affected.

Illness as Servant

Many children learn from an early age that illness can gain attention. A parent will often comfort a child in pain and at its worst a child will pretend pain and cry for attention. As an adult, we may have an unconscious memory of being comforted when we were ill as a child. Having something wrong with us is a legitimate reason for gaining attention - love and concern, extra help and companionship.

One evening, after reading her a bedtime story, my daughter (aged 6) suddenly asked: "Daddy, if I was really ill and couldn't travel in the car, would I have to stay here?" Our daughter lived with my wife 106 miles away and they were visiting in one of the school holidays. She had enjoyed her visit and I was due to return them home the next day. I was taken aback by her question but managed to respond quickly: "If you were too ill to go by car, I'd hire a helicopter and fly you home." This seemed to do the trick and I knew she would still be fit and healthy in the morning.

This incident graphically illustrated to me the potential for using illness to maintain or gain a desired situation. I was simply stunned at how early this connection with health and desired outcome was so cleverly demonstrated - not to mention the extraordinary application of logic that children employ.

The society many of us experience, particularly in the western world, has become a lot less tactile and more separate over the years. People are busy looking after their own interests and time spent with children has been replaced with extra toys, television, and video games. Like all humans, we try things out until we gain the feedback for the result we are looking for. Unfortunately for many of us, this feedback becomes linked with how successfully we can manipulate our well-being.

You might think that my focus on children doesn't apply to you as an adult, but stop and think of any time when you have perhaps used illness for gaining attention - whether it be from someone you want a show of love from, or simply to demonstrate your unique special condition. The rarer you can make your illness, the more special you feel! The long-term problem with this is that you may find it difficult to reverse what you have created. This is when illness takes control of you, rather than you having control of it.

At this point, many of you may be protesting, saying things like, 'I don't need attention! That doesn't apply to my situation. I am genuinely ill and I don't want sympathy from anyone!'

If that is the case, ask yourself this: Why do you think you are ill?

Okay, here's another example of using illness. In much of society, illness is the only legitimate reason not to have to do something; whether it is work-related or leisure-related. It's no use phoning the boss and saying you've decided not to go into work because you don't feel like it today! But if you explain instead that you are too ill to go to work, the boss simply wishes you a quick recovery and tells you to come back as soon as you are better.

In the first example, you could jeopardise your job. In the second example your circumstances are accepted as 'one of those things that can happen to us all'.

Mind over Matter

The power of suggestion works at many levels. For example, just imagine for a moment cutting a lemon in half and sinking your teeth into the juicy fruit. The usual response here is to notice how your saliva glands are activated and your mouth begins to water. If this example doesn't do it for you, think about anything that causes you to experience sexual arousal. Notice the responses in your physical body, simply brought about by focusing your thoughts on an imagined activity.

Now ask yourself this. If such a reaction can be obtained simply by thinking about a citrus fruit or a sexual fantasy, how might your body respond to other thoughts you have?

Try it! Focus your mind on your stomach or the taste in your mouth - and start feeling a bit sick! Just think: 'I don't feel too good'. Don't dwell on this! Now think: 'I feel really good'.

With the above fresh in your mind, let's take a closer look at some of the ways we may make ourselves ill. Once you have looked at some of the things that can cause illness, consider those things I have mentioned that will help you to regain a healthy state - or even not become ill in the first place! Believe it or not, the choice is yours.

There are many reasons why people become ill. Here are a few:

- Guilt - feeling that you deserve to be punished
- Stress - inability to cope with a life situation
- Unworthiness - believing that you don't deserve to be healthy
- Expectation - there's something going around I am bound to catch it
- Belief in illness - everyone gets ill at some time in their lives
- Attention - I want someone to love me
- Powerlessness - I can become ill and someone will have to save me
- Excuse to get out of a situation - I don't like working here anymore - I don't want to visit so and so
- History - everyone on this side of my family gets this
- Inevitability - we all get old and older people get things going wrong with them - bodies deteriorate!

Most of us are full of the expectation that illness can strike us at any time and that we have no power or control over it. Our focus is on worry and concern for our well-being rather than joy of the moment and happiness in our current health. We constantly bemoan our circumstances and plan for rainy days whenever we can. Illness is acceptable in our society as a legitimate reason for not being present somewhere. It is an easy option to extricate ourselves from aspects of life we find stressful. Saying you are ill is easier than admitting you do not wish to participate. Telling someone you 'just don't want to' never seems to be enough. Telling someone you are ill is accepted with little question.

Symptoms as Messages

Quite often, we will first realise something is different or 'wrong' when we experience a physical symptom - any sensation or change in body function or a visual physical difference. A typical example might be an ache or pain somewhere. However, a backache or shoulder ache may not just relate to a poor posture. It can indicate that circumstances or situations have become burdensome to us. Other physical symptoms may indicate the way we have aired our feelings about someone or some thing - 'pain in the neck!'

Consider the statements you make about yourself and others. Are you using expressions that could cause you to exhibit physical symptoms? Be aware of the clichés you use:

- It's getting me down
- I'd give my right arm for...
- I'm fed up with...
- It's a pain in the...

And so on...

Stress

This has to be my number one favourite illness generator. It has so much potential I'm surprised we don't make it either a statutory requirement to ensure our misery or a national treasure to show off to others!

Like most people, I have experienced physical symptoms from stressful situations. And stress can be anything from problems at home or work to problems with relationships and life circumstances.

Some years ago, I manifested a physical ailment just by being in the regular presence of someone whom I found challenging company. Once this person left, the ailment left too! By dealing with the stress, physical ailments subside or completely disappear. (I should like to add here that the solution isn't necessarily to banish people from your close proximity - that example was merely to illustrate a stressful situation only realised with hindsight).

Monitoring
You can usefully monitor physical discomfort as a measure of your ability to alter a stressful situation. Humans are very cleverly designed to have these built-in barometers to give us feedback.

I am not going to espouse an exhaustive list of the many ways you might be able to alleviate stress through spiritual practices such as meditation or relaxation therapies - I leave that to you. Suffice to say there are some benefits to be had from these. All I am hoping to achieve is to provide another perspective on health.

It is also worth mentioning here, that when you begin to take charge of your health and well-being, symptoms and circumstances may persist or become apparently worse. See this positively, as the body adjusting to the new reality. Old cells or infections have to be removed. The body knows how to do this safely.

Body Awareness

Let's take aches and pains… try and locate what you are doing to create some of them. You may find that many are avoidable. As a teenager at school, I often endured frequent headaches. Part of this was the lighting and the stuffy atmosphere in the classroom, but much of it resulted from my seating position and general posture. After a bit of experimentation, I realised that I could feel pressure points developing and by shifting my position slightly, now and again throughout the lesson, my headaches diminished considerably.

Turning Things Around

Try to foster a deep belief that you expect to be healthy. This should be both your goal and your condition. The only reason you should want to be ill in the future is so you can remember what it was like! Stop using illness as an option to solve other problems in your life.

Try communicating with every cell in your body. Inform your cells that they are working well for you, and you would like them to maintain your good health at every level.

Reluctance of Others to Accept Your Changes

People around you become used to you being a certain way. If you try to alter the way you are, some people will embrace the change, while others will feel uncomfortable and have a tendency to pressure you to remain the person they are familiar with. Indeed, you may also feel uncomfortable exhibiting your new behaviour and/or beliefs in front of people who know the 'old you' very well. It's difficult to explain this situation of changing nature. I will try to illustrate the point with some more examples.

Perhaps, in the past, you have been an argumentative person and now realise the error of your ways. You approach someone who is familiar with the 'old you', intending to be quite pleasant, only to be confronted by the sort of defensive reaction that would have been levelled at the 'old you'!

Equally, you may find that you fall back into old patterns of behaviour when you are in the company of particular people. A common example is seen in parent and child relationships, where a child (now an adult) visits the parent/s and complies with what he/she thinks is expected by the parent, or where both parties revert to behaviour that existed in previous family life together.

In relation to health, the person who is ill may start to tell people that he/she is improving. In response to this, someone may be dismissive of this apparent improvement and even suggest that the person is not being realistic about their condition - which will undoubtedly revert to its previous state.

Try not to be put off by these situations when they arise. It is important for you to continue with the beliefs that you personally want to build on.

The Deeper Perspective

Healing Technique
There are a number of different views held by people on healing and the various 'do's' and 'don'ts' etc. Every healer develops his/her own techniques and discovers the things that work best for him/her self and his/her clients. Let's consider a few things that you might come across.

Personal Beliefs and Personal Reality
Firstly, please reflect on the notion of beliefs creating reality. Secondly, what follows is only an indicator of beliefs held by some practitioners and not intended as a set-in-stone explanation of what to expect or believe in. You choose what you believe. However, when you are starting to develop your skills in healing, you will undoubtedly come across varying views held by people already practising healing. Some people will warn you against certain practices and many will say that there are only certain ways of accomplishing healing in the right way. By all

means consider their views, but always ask yourself: "What feels right to me?"

Working with the Client

The first time you meet a potential client, you may not appear to do much in the way of obvious healing practice at all. To begin with, you simply talk with the person. The reason for this is twofold: to put them at ease and to pick up as many clues and as much information as possible about the nature of the injury or illness you have been asked to help cure. It is important to look beyond the symptoms of illness, examining life-style, personal attitudes, and core beliefs[8].

As you listen to the client, you may pick up on terms such as, 'a part of me feels...' or 'I had a feeling...' etc. Others might include: 'When I was a child...' or 'Someone once told me...' These expressions give a useful insight into the unconscious condition of the individual and the beliefs they are acting on. Techniques that use these clues as part of therapy are encompassed in practices such as Core Transformation[9] and NLP (Neuro-Linguistic Programming).[10] Both practices share some common elements and are closely related in their aims and outcomes. There are other techniques, but it is not in the remit of this book to cover them in detail.

Quite often, simply through allowing a person to talk about him/her self - with a little guidance through specific questions on my part, I have witnessed healing starting to take place before my eyes. Using the Crystal Wand now becomes much more effective. Energy is able to go to where it is needed and the

---

[8] Core beliefs are essentially unconscious beliefs that you have about your life and reality. Regardless of what you do in life, core beliefs work in the background and directly affect the life you lead.

[9] Core Transformation refers to changing deeply held unconscious beliefs that affect our lives in many different ways.

[10] NLP is about reprogramming the unconscious beliefs we hold about ourselves to improve the way we function in our daily personal lives.

psychological blocks for healing to take place have been diminished or removed. There is little point in attempting to heal someone if they are rigidly holding onto beliefs that maintain the 'negative' condition they experience.

Some conditions will change completely in an instant. Other conditions may take a little time to show improvement. One view held, is that it takes time to put energy into a condition that becomes manifest in your physical reality and because of this, it may take time to reverse or change that condition. Some of this is also linked to our view of reality. Time is physically perceived as a serialised set of events. However, it is simultaneous in terms of the universe. Because of this, there is no reason why we should not experience instant changes in our reality. We are only limited by our own beliefs in the reality we feel comfortable experiencing. Total faith and 'knowing' outside of our 'comfort zones'[11] is not a feeling most people are used to having. The example below attempts to illustrate the difference between believing and knowing.

The Importance of Knowing

Consider two common activities. We reach for our cup of tea or coffee, grab the cup and lift it to our lips to drink. We are in no doubt that we will achieve the objective of having a sip of the liquid - because we know that we will. The action of drinking is one that we have performed many times and there is no need to question it. If I simply believed that I would be able to take a drink, this would leave open the possibility for doubt. Belief is not the same as knowing. For most able-bodied people, rising to stand from a sitting position is equally as normal. We neither, consciously plough through the mental process of deciding how we should best stand, or consider for one moment that we might not be able to stand. We simply stand.

---

[11] Comfort Zones - In general, we will go only to places where we feel safe and secure. This can be both mental and physical.

The above example illustrates the feeling we must achieve as a healer. When you know beyond belief and doubt that healing works - you will never have to question it.

Empathy
At one level it is possible to become so empathic with someone else's condition that you actually begin to take on symptoms yourself. Although the symptoms may not develop into the actual condition suffered by the client, you might experience some physical discomfort. I personally find it helps to remain fairly neutral - in so far as I am totally impartial to any particular outcome. Besides which, you are not focusing healing energy to decide on whether someone recovers or not. You are focusing energy to enable it to work in whatever way is most appropriate to helping the client.

Sometimes a client will not recover, but the healing may ease their discomfort and even help transition to be smoother at the point of physical death. The important thing here is not to feel bad about your efforts or disillusioned with any healing you have been trying. Everyone has to go sometime and the choice may not be one that you are in a position to influence.

Resonance
In addition to empathy, it is possible to resonate with a client's condition. A similar ailment in you, and known to you, or possibly an ailment or condition you have heard about that you feel drawn towards, may be brought into your awareness. Put another way, a concern about a similar condition existing in (or potentially coming to exist in) your own body may trigger that condition. In healing - and you will have to excuse the description here as I have to present the ideas in a three-dimensional visual construct - you can choose to use energy from yourself - projected through yourself, or from outside of yourself - direct from the universal energy field.[12] Traditionally, healers claim to channel healing

---

[12] The Universal Energy Field permeates the whole universe. It is sentient consciousness from which everything is manifest. Other names for the field

energy through their own bodies - directing the energy to where it is most needed. I personally prefer not to heal in this way (except on some occasions when healing my own body) and instead focus energy directly from the universal energy field. Channelling through, or from, your own body can also leave you feeling a bit tired or emotionally drained. Healers who use this method often have a glass of water before and after a healing session. Part of this is symbolic ritual and part of it can prevent you getting a headache.

Sensations
Sometimes, when you are healing a person they will report feeling certain sensations or temperature changes. This is quite normal. However, it is worth mentioning to your client before you begin the actual healing process, that physical sensations may also be felt. Generally, the healing you undertake will be mostly non-contact. However, sometimes the client may believe that you are stroking or pressing on their body in the areas you are working on or near. I mention this partly as a word of caution, particularly if you are, for example, a man working with a female client. Sometimes, having another person present can be helpful in observing the healing session. This of course is not always possible - although it does offer reassurance to someone who thinks he/she may have been physically touched when in fact no contact has taken place. I often suggest to a client that he/she may keep their eyes open, or if closed, open them whenever he/she feels a need to see what is happening.

Personal Action Intervention (PAI)
Put simply, this is my label for taking personal control over your condition and intervening in the illness process by deciding to have your situation improve. Personal Action Intervention can take any number of forms, but at its most basic, you simply decide that you will be better and will recover.

---

include: Sentient Power Field, Unified Field and Zero-Point Field

Other forms of Personal Action Intervention include employing things that reinforce your belief in your improvement. One example could be modifying your diet to introduce foods that you believe can give you a stronger ability to fight disease. Another example might be to create your own healing ritual. Alternatively, verbal affirmations that you are feeling healthier every day may help. Whatever form of Personal Action Intervention you decide upon, know that it is going to benefit you. If you choose something that doesn't seem to help, simply find an alternative method that you can believe in. It really doesn't matter what you choose - although I would avoid something that is linked to, or could become, a personal superstition - that is to say, do not place your belief in something such as, wearing a talisman that keeps you healthy - just in case you forget to wear it one day and become ill. Having said this, when you get an improvement in health that is the outcome you desire - regardless of how it occurs.

If your Personal Action Intervention involves tackling unhelpful, unconscious beliefs, try using NLP or writing down your thoughts and feelings on paper. Try having a conversation with yourself or with a higher aspect of your being - or with another being altogether! Write down your questions and write down the answers that you receive. At first you will think all the answers are just you deciding what they should be. However, if you let go of controlling this and write down the first thing that comes into your head, you'll be amazed at what you start to produce.

Probable Outcomes
There is a theory that we live in a universe of multiple possibilities. Another way to view this, is to say that there are several probable outcomes in any situation. For example, one outcome is that we become ill. Another outcome is that we remain healthy. Every time that you have a thought about something, you set up a probable event leading to a possible outcome. In scientific terms, you live in a quantum universe where nothing is truly predictable.

Now consider two more situations:

- I knock a ceramic cup off the table and it falls on a hard tiled floor and breaks.

- I knock a ceramic cup off the table and it falls on a hard tiled floor and remains undamaged.

The only difference between these last two events was my expectation of knowing what was going to happen. In both examples, my sense of knowing the outcome was equally strong. However, this in itself was based on my personal state of well-being and general outlook on life. Both events had opposing probable outcomes. At one moment the outcome was perfectly balanced. It was only at the point where I changed the balance that one probable outcome occurred over the other in my experience of physical reality.

So how did I influence the outcome? The event took place in an instant. I had no real time as I perceived it, to think about what I was going to believe the outcome would be. In both examples I went into an automatic response based on my state of my being in that moment. The outcome was perfect in relation to my beliefs about dropped cups and hard tiled floors.

There is however, in my experience, a caveat to include here. You can change reality in every moment of your existence and you can change an outcome if you choose to do so. It is therefore perfectly possible to know that ceramic cups falling on hard tiled floors will break and at the same time know that they do not always have to break. You can make a choice about any perceived outcome in your life - whether to accept or change a situation. The difficulty arises when you put blocks in the way - consciously or unconsciously. A conscious block may be a thought that something cannot happen. An unconscious block might be that we have a fear of the unknown.

The Universal Energy Field

The universal energy field has been given many labels, including the Sentient Power Field (Eugene Halliday)[13] and the Zero Point Field (Lynne McTaggart).[14] Put simply, this is a field of conscious energy that joins and permeates all things in the universe. As Seth[15] says, everything has conscious awareness of everything else in the universe.

My preferred description of the field is that offered by Eugene Halliday, below. However, it sometimes takes a few reads to get your head around what is being described!

"A field of pure sentience that permeates the universe, experiencing all of its self-initiated motion patterns simultaneously and at equal stress. Where a super-stress is placed on a given form or forms [already in simultaneous existence but not seen as separate], the state of consciousness becomes non-simultaneous and non immediate. In consciousness, the forms are serialised and therefore apprehended only one at a time. (This gives us the sense of experiencing something in a linear space-time way). Wherever a super-stress is placed on a form in the field it in turn super-stresses other forms to maintain a balanced tension in the field. After the introduction of super-stress into the power field, pure sentience is overlapped by the serialising process of formal presentation. The serialisation process is the precondition of what we call consciousness. In it the forms, which had previously been in simultaneous relation in the pure sentience, are precipitated into serialisation - presented one after another. This is the generation of the time process.

The simultaneity of the equally stressed forms of the sentient power field is called Eternity. The serialisation of these forms is

---

[13] Eugene Halliday - Wrote about the Sentient Power Field in a booklet called 'Truth' - published by the International Hermeneutic Society, Clwyd, Wales.
[14] Wrote a book called The Field and runs conferences on The Field
[15] Refer to the Seth books by Jane Roberts

called Time. Eternity holds simultaneously what Time presents serially.

Every element wrenched from Eternity by Time, lapses back into eternity on the removal of the temporal super-stress."

Another way of perhaps understanding this is to consider the possibility that nothing exists until we realise it through our senses. When our senses are no longer focusing on something, it no longer exists to us in our physical reality.[16]

The reason I mention the field is that we can tune into various aspects of it to help with our healing. One aspect is that it enables us to do absent healing. Another aspect is that we can focus energy from the field to produce a change in state to promote healing of both the etheric and physical bodies. We can also use the field to travel through time and have an experience of simultaneous existence - awareness of being in more than one place or time. This can help with changing a past experience from our relative position in the present - which in turn alters our negative perception of an experience that may be affecting our state of health now. There are many other wonderful qualities of the field but these are not aspects I am going to focus on here.

Absent Healing
It is possible to send healing to someone, even if they are several hundred miles away. A possible reason for this is the connection that all consciousness has with itself throughout the universal sentient energy field. If you know the person, hold an image of him/her in mind and imagine you are going through a healing process as if he/she is with you in person. You can imagine healing with your Wand, or you might like to try the following:

---

[16] ibid footnote 13

Cup your hands in front of you and focus all of your attention on them. Imagine that a ball of blue healing light is forming in your cupped hands. When you can see this, add some red sparks of fire, emanating from all around the blue ball of energy. Now, gently launch the ball from your hands and see it travel away from you towards the person you are healing. See the blue ball propelled by its red fire and watch it go to and envelop the person you are healing.

If you do not know the person you are healing, you can either ask for a photograph of the person or simply think of their name while you perform your healing exercise.

Ruby Laser
In order to give you some idea of how the crystal wand may operate, I will compare it to the principle behind a ruby laser - the first type of laser invented around 1960. A flash tube around a ruby crystal excites the electrons in the ruby, amplifying and accelerating them between a mirrored and partially mirrored surface, until a pure beam of red light is emitted from the partially silvered end.

Electrons can be bumped up to higher energy levels by the injection of energy, i.e. by a flash of light. When an electron drops from an outer to an inner level, 'excess' energy is given off as light. The wavelength or colour of the emitted light is precisely related to the amount of energy released.

A characteristic of laser light is that it is coherent. That is, the emitted light waves are in phase with one another and are so nearly parallel that they can travel for long distances without spreading. (In contrast, incoherent light from a light bulb diffuses in all directions). Coherence means that laser light can be focused with great precision. Indeed, laser applications are already used in the medical field.

Imagine now, that your hand around the shaft of the wand represents the flash tube in the laser description. As you send energy through your hand, electrons in the wand are excited and photons are released and accelerated inside the shaft. As they reach an increased level of activity, photons pass through and out of the crystal. At the same time, focused energy from the sentient field permeates the wand and helps to direct the photons through the crystal. The focus of the healer in knowing that the right energy will leave the wand is enough to draw on the necessary and desired qualities of the field.

Photonic Healing
When I first decided on the term 'Photonic Healing' I was considering the process that might be occurring in the crystal wand. I postulated that it was possible to affect energy with thought (manipulating consciousness units[17] in the sentient field) and synthesise that energy with electrons and photons. Photonic healing is then, the synthesis of photons with the sentient energy field through creative visualisation producing transformative light that can effect healing at both an etheric field and physical cellular level.

Missing Antimatter
Another of my theories may, I admit, be entirely incorrect. However, I have often wondered whether the missing antimatter in the universe is in fact all around us in quantum miniscule particles - bombarding our physical bodies and cells constantly. A particle [electron] and its antimatter particle [positron] annihilate when they meet.

A change in our well-being reduces the effectiveness of some of our cells to not be affected by this constant positron bombardment, and as a result our physical matter is damaged - perhaps causing the symptoms of cancer or even contributing to the aging process. By using PAI and Photonic Healing, it may be

---

[17] Consciousness Units - a term coined by Seth in the Jane Roberts books to describe the tiniest units of consciousness - the building blocks of the universe

possible that cells are given a renewed capacity to resist positron bombardment. I have previously tried to find someone to discuss this idea with me, but at the time of writing, no one has come forward to either prove or disprove this line of thinking.

The importance of creating reality in relation to health

Beliefs - The Root of Reality
Seth explains that "physical data will always seem to reinforce beliefs and our beliefs form the reality we experience"[18]. In relation to my discourse on healing, your sense of health and well-being is caused by your beliefs. In broad terms, if you believe your condition is making you unhappy, it will, and the unhappiness will then reinforce the condition. Everyone has within them the ability to change their ideas about reality and about themselves. "No one can change your beliefs for you, nor can they be forced upon you from without. However, you can change them for yourself"[19]. A simple example of this could be the advice a parent might bestow on a child. The child may rebel against the advice, seeing it as an imposed limitation against their motivation, and do things their own way. At a future time, as older child or adult, the individual may choose to view or experience a similar situation differently and be willing to voluntarily change their own belief about it.

Again, Seth restates, "there is no karma to be paid off as punishment unless you believe that there are crimes for which you must pay"[20]. However, it may be difficult for some of you to accept this, due to 'root assumptions'[21] of the society and reality you inhabit.

Root Assumptions - Mass Beliefs

---

[18] The Nature of Personal Reality
[19] ibid footnote 18
[20] ibid footnote 18
[21] Each system of reality has its own set of agreements.

Regardless of any personal beliefs that you hold - consciously or otherwise - the society and the world of which you are a member has evolved many of its own collective beliefs. These beliefs are sometimes referred to as root assumptions. For example, we accept that night follows day, gravity holds us down, and so on.

Root assumptions have been developed by our collective societies for thousands of years. That is to say, we are accepting of some commonly held beliefs as being fixed facts in our existence. The science fiction writer, Brian Aldiss illustrated this in an interesting way in his book 'Cryptozoic'. In this story, some people mind-travel back in history. Although they have a real awareness of where they go to, they cannot completely interact with the world that they are in. They never make complete tactile contact with the ground and they can pass through many objects. However, if an object is very old and well-established, it has a density that cannot be passed through. I am not saying that Brian Aldiss was thinking along these lines, but his creative observation lends itself very well to the notion that established beliefs over many years have more substance than beliefs appearing more recently [accepting a serialised physical reality time structure].

Psychosomatic Illness

There was a time when illness, deemed to have no apparent legitimacy and brought on by an individual's thoughts, was labelled psychosomatic. I remember this term being used a lot around the late 1970s and early 1980s. Put simply, symptoms arising from neurosis [in the mind] about situations or circumstances. However, in terms of creating our own view of perceived physical reality, psychosomatic illness could produce all the physical symptoms of a recognisable set of ailments. I do recall though, that to accuse someone of having a psychosomatic illness was often used as being dismissive of the individual's complaint. Looking at this label now, I see it as a precursor to manifesting a physical condition of ill health.

Placebo Effect

Telling someone that something will work can have an effect on his/her health. One reason for this is the reprogramming of reality through a change in personal belief. At some level, you created your ailment by focusing on it in the first place - either through self-talk or visualisation, etc. A person whom you perceive as being able to help you can actually reverse the effect of your former belief by offering positive suggestion in a way that you can accept as being authentic. This kicks your positive belief into action and you change your reality because you expect to improve.

The way you are thinking, and what you expect, produces chemical changes in the brain. The role of the healer is a key factor. Enthusiasm, belief and commitment that the client finds compelling, and the way it is conveyed, can make a huge difference to the restoration of health.

The Paradox

Because you can create a reality where you bring personal illness into being, it then becomes physically manifest in the world of other people who share a belief in those possibilities. In this world, root assumptions exist and people agree on shared experiences of reality. Some people become so involved in this reality that they become illness specialists i.e. doctors, nurses, and surgeons. This is an example of how physical reality operates once creative thought becomes manifest. As we manifest individual and collective realities, other people come forward to either reinforce that requirement in us, or help to maintain balance in physical reality once it is made manifest. As we see with our eyes and hear with our ears - and in general receive information through our five physical senses - we reinforce physical reality in our own way. Collectively, many of us agree on aspects of reality and these become even more fixed in place. Change may often only occur en masse when our collective consciousness changes and this is often brought about by exceptional individuals with a clarity of vision not bound by existing [created] physicality.

Most people lack mental discipline and have little ability to focus concentrated attention for long. One result of this is that free-flowing sloppiness gives the impression that reality appears to simply 'be here or there' and there is little anyone can do to alter it much. Our focus on what we see and experience is based on our choices of whether we 'like' or 'dislike' something and we move around in a comparative physical world - picking and choosing within the parameters of our beliefs about reality. A problem with this approach is the way we create many things that we do not realise we have created!

Summary
I don't intend to write one of those long essay-type conclusions here. However, I think it is worth reiterating some of the key points made in this book.

Be conscious of the messages you give to yourself or send to others. Consider how you feel about yourself, other people, and the things in life that appear to affect you.

Notice when any aches or pains occur and consider whether you may have contributed to, or created, them in some way.

Ask yourself: Does illness or a general lack of physical well-being serve any purpose for me?

Consider that sometimes, illness is used to attract attention, gain affection, or help us to [legitimately] avoid doing something.

Sometimes we become so absorbed or stressed about our working lives, that we feel unable to take time out for ourselves in case things go wrong in our absence. An illness or injury may force us to stop working and spend more time relaxing.

The way you think about your health directly affects the experience of health that you have. If you are ill, rather than focusing attention on the illness, focus on how it will feel to be better. This is not a form of denial. Accept and embrace your illness, but decide that every day you will become increasingly healthy. Have intent to recover and most importantly, 'expect' good health.

Notice what you say to people and pass on as fact. Notice what you hear people saying to you and about other people and events as fact. Question what you think you know.

Ask yourself: "What do I believe?" When you answer this question, ask another: "How do I know what I know?" And finally: "What evidence do I really have that what I Know has truth?"

Finally, I hope that this book has given you some new ideas about healing and how you can maintain health. Some of the things I have mentioned may need further exploration and some things may present a challenge to your current beliefs and ways of thinking. Whatever your views, be open to new possibilities. Know that you can make a difference both to yourself and others. Your ability to heal without the help of doctors and medicines will one day soon become very useful.

I will leave the last word on Crystal Wand Healing, to a friend:

"I do a lot of building restoration work and my thumb had been playing up for years. I was very sceptical about the wand but was amazed! I felt a slight electrical tingly feeling and it's been perfect ever since. It definitely works".

Phil, West Sussex

Other work by Richard Gentle:

How we perform negative miracles

Quantum Mass Superstructures - creating the world you experience

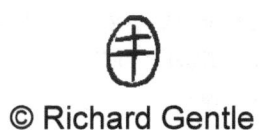

© Richard Gentle

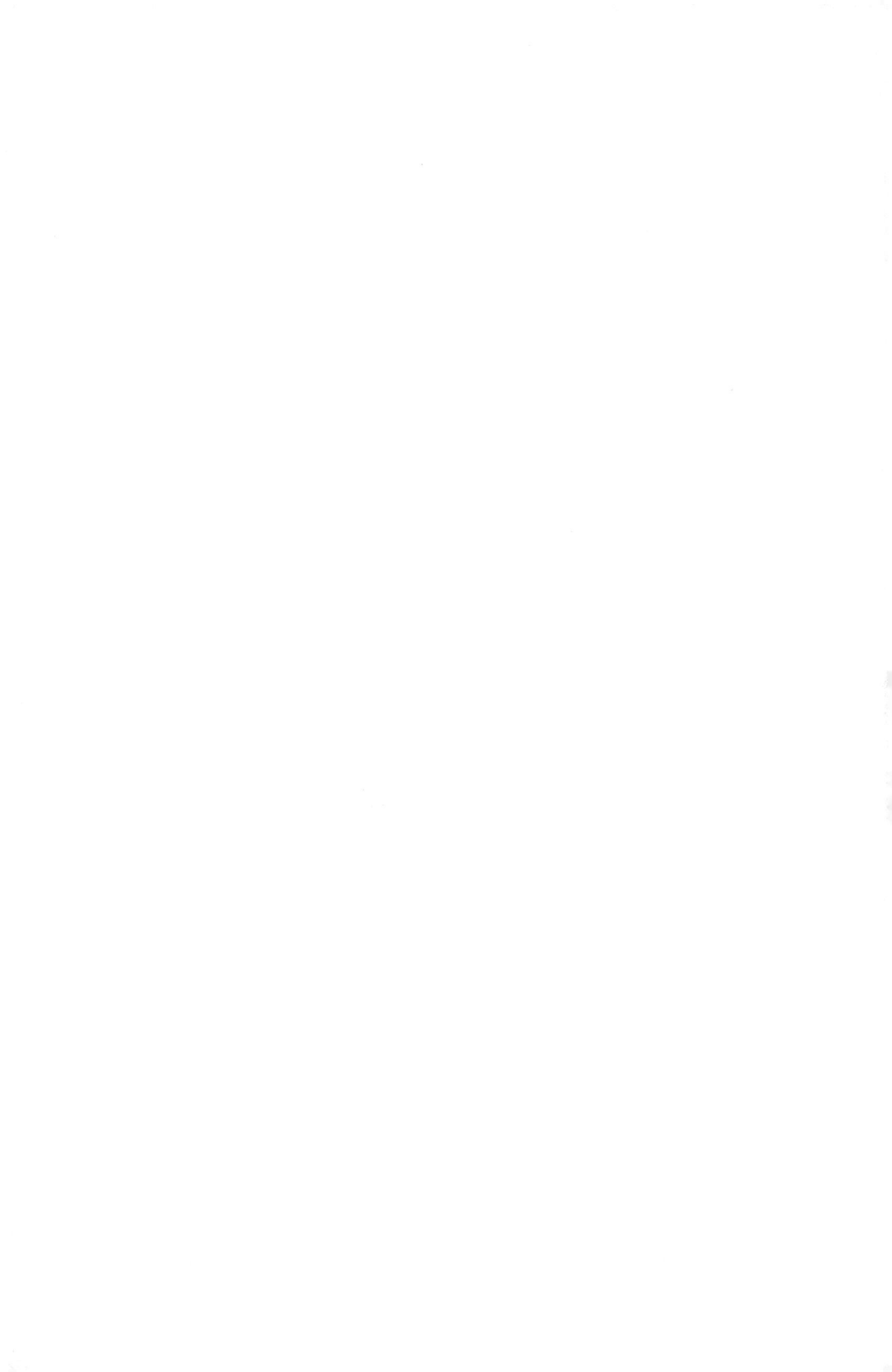

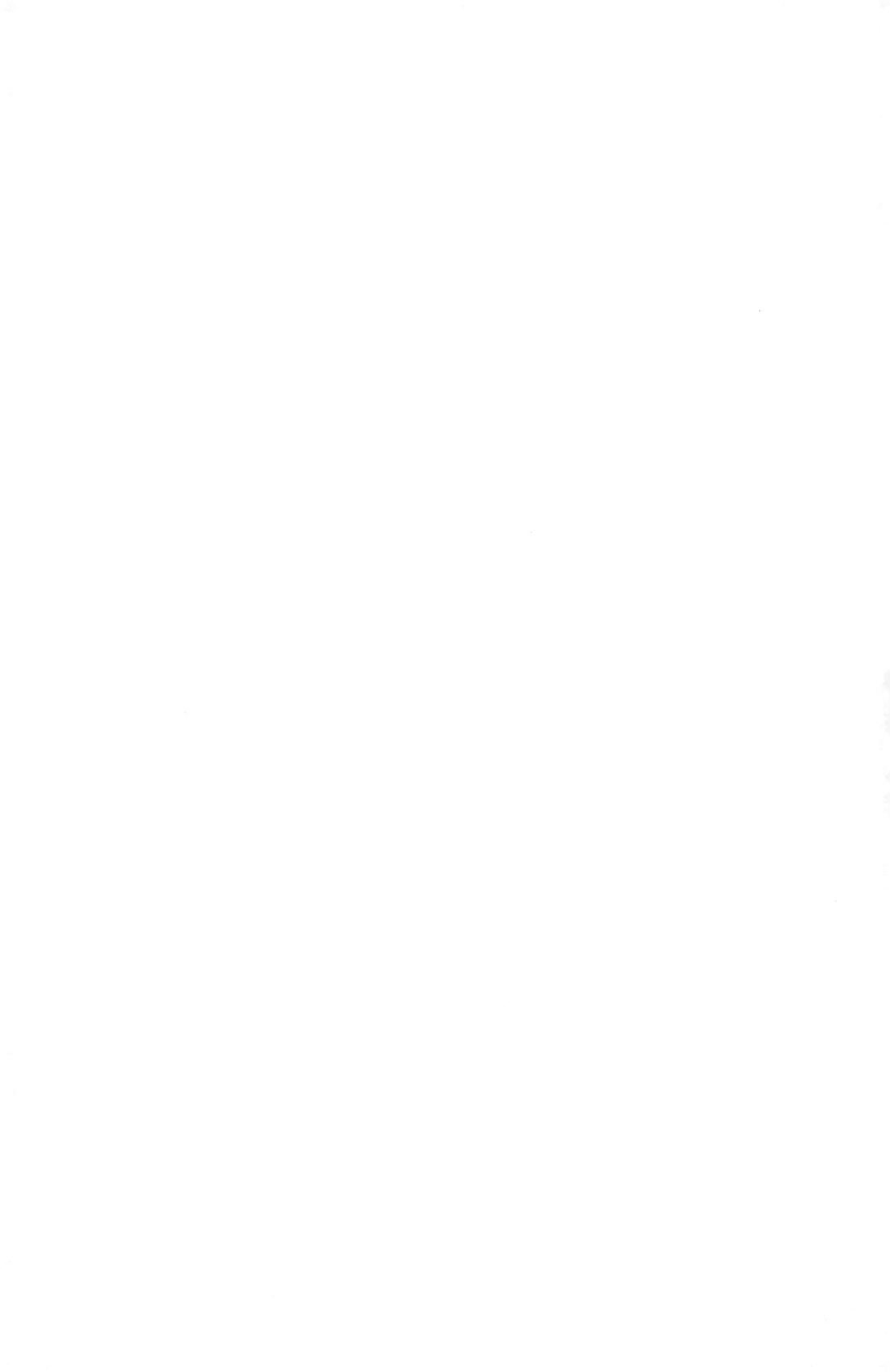

www.ingramcontent.com/pod-product-compliance
Lightning Source LLC
Chambersburg PA
CBHW061219280526
45784CB00006B/2545